How To Give A Great Presentation

And

Love Your Audience

How to give a great presentation and love your audience. Is a book for anyone who has to deliver a message, tell a story - or speak to another human being. Most of us are quite relaxed and confident when we're with our friends and family. We can tell a story or even tell a joke. But put us on a platform and we can feel very different. When we speak to an audience, we often put on a public mask … and use a different voice. Why can't we seem to be ourselves when we give a talk?

In this book, we will look at all aspects of spoken communication, from structure right through to delivery. We will learn how to have a conversation with our audience - to be ourselves - so that we connect with them every time we speak. In a few simple steps, you can learn to be a confident and authentic public speaker. There are specific exercises to build a more confident you in preparation for your speech.

Whether you're a CEO presenting to shareholders, an entrepreneur promoting your business, a manager motivating your team, a creative pitching an idea, a charity worker asking for donations or a parent speaking at your son's wedding, this book will help you become a confident and authentic public speaker, so that when you speak, your audience will listen. And, hopefully, you'll enjoy the experience too.

There are helpful tips and activities for the reader to try, and summaries of what to do for each stage of developing a presentation.

The Author:- Gary Sellors

Gary is a certified NLP Trainer, trained personally by Dr John Grinder (NLP Co-creator & Professor of Linguistics). Gary is a much sort after person in the business world, recognised and used by many top companies now, and therefore able to offer a whole range of skills to the development of people in the many businesses.

Gary is CIPD Qualified with an HR and Management background, Also a tutor for the London College of Clinical Hypnosis and a YMCA Personal Fitness Trainer. Along with good knowledge of Emotional Intelligence, Quantum Touch, Thought Field Therapy, Animal Healing, Reiki and EFT.

He has previously done training and developing with the likes of the CLRPG (Central London Retail Personnel Group) which includes the likes of Harrods, Marks & Spencer's, Harvey Nichol's, Elstree Film Studios, etc.. Using his experience and passion for the training and development of Directors / Managers and Sports Professionals at all levels. Including coaching top athletes on their mindset and helping them win British and European Gold medals.

He offers bespoke training in many areas for businesses and one to one coaching along with a massive range of therapy work, along with continuing his work on restoring Natural Eyesight, by working with the brain and a few simple exercises in retraining the eyes.

Business Coaching

Presentation Skills

With

Gary Sellors

An excellent presentation has never been more important. At work, we are constantly aware of the need to keep customers on board, persuade staff or influence peers.

You want me to do what... A speech takes a step-at-a-time approach to develop a belting presentation, from unpicking the original brief, understanding just what an audience wants and constructing compelling content that will keep them rapt with attention. With anecdotes and expert input, covers all the essentials necessary to make a good presentation, including advice on how to build confidence; increase personal competence; use body language; maximise the effectiveness of room layout; use technology and implement disaster recovery methods.

Together with key learning points and top tips, You want me to do what... A speech is essential reading for anyone who wants to exude confidence and nail that presentation.

Business Coaching

How To Give A Great Presentation

And

Love Your Audience

Contents

Anxiety (How to Remove)

Top Tips for presenting

Tips for using flip charts

Impromptu speaking

Welcome

Presenting powerfully

Your sense of yourself affects the way you present

You develop your own style and make your own 'rules' being more of who you are.

The content of your presentation is secondary to whom you are when presenting.

Your enthusiasm for the subject matter is important.

Presenting powerfully requires you to be yourself rather than add on extra's

Who do you know is a great presenter?

For me, I would choose –

Sir Alex Ferguson.

Sir Alexander Chapman Ferguson CBE is a Scottish former football manager and player who managed Manchester United from 1986 to 2013. He is regarded to be one of the greatest and most successful managers of all time. Ferguson played as a forward for several Scottish clubs, including Dunfermline Athletic and Rangers.

I have had the privilege to meet Sir Alex at Wembley Stadium in my Medical role. Sir Alex Ferguson for me. It was always how

he could keep control of the Manchester United team, dealing

with the world press and just winning so much over the many years of his management.

Michael Schumacher.

Michael Schumacher is a retired German racing driver who raced in Formula One for Jordan Grand Prix, Benetton and Ferrari, where he spent the majority of his career, as well as for Mercedes upon his return to the sport.

I have always been amazed how focused Michael was when he had a bad race, of which he never had many. The way he presented to the interviews as he left the car. Was to always say, it was about the next race, never did he had time for reflecting on the past.

A great mindset. I would have loved to have read his own autobiography written by him in his own words. Sadly, this may now never happen. Latest news on the recovery of Michael Schumacher, having had a ski accident in 2013. Michael is still in recovery and lives by Lake Geneva.

Think about great presenters you admire. List 3 things

1.

2.

3.

What is it you like about them?

1.

2.

3.

What do you enjoy about them?

1.

2.

3.

What makes you remember them the most?

1.

2.

3.

What makes them that way?

1.

2.

3.

Behavioural Modelling – What is it?

Behavioural modelling in NLP or Neuro-Linguistic Programming is the study of how people get delightful and successful results in their lives - and how people get less-than-welcome results, too.

So, at its simplest, NLP Behavioural Modelling is the study of what accounts for the results that people achieve. In other words, what are the thoughts, behaviours, skills, beliefs, values, and other attitudinal qualities that they use to do what they do?

For example, Behavioural Modelling can be used to discover the 'mechanics' of thinking, feeling and behaving like an excellent football player or a mediocre teacher utilise to produce their performance.

Why use behavioural modelling?

In very simple modelling you can learn from/about someone else by asking lots of questions and by very carefully listening to and observing their replies. In doing so you are likely to make some useful discoveries - such as that they prepare themselves in a particular manner or that they have a certain way of recovering from setbacks.

You may be able to incorporate some of their methods into your own behavioural repertoire or even find their interest in their subject so contagious that you also want to take up the activity.

The other person, too, can benefit from your modelling. Many people take their skills for granted. When you ask detailed questions about a person's strategy for doing something they

may come to recognise just how skilful they are.

As you obtain details of their strategy you may discover areas

for improvement and alert them to these.

By learning to model with precision and skill you can pass on

the behaviour, or part of it, to others.

In modelling a person's behaviour you temporarily enter their Model of the World. Doing this increases your understanding of them. This is especially so when you model a person's way of having feelings.

Through self-modelling, you discover more about your own feelings, thoughts and behaviours. This is a particularly important application of behavioural modelling.

For example, you can discover the Anchors to which you 'automatically' respond, the way you use your five senses, how you use your self-talk, how you use your body - and how do each of these contributes towards the feelings you experience.

Presenting yourself - How would you present yourself?

What is a presentation?

A presentation is a means of communication which can be adapted to various speaking situations, such as talking to a group, addressing a meeting or briefing a team. To be effective, step-by-step preparation and the method and means of presenting the information should be carefully considered.

If you were to introduce yourself to someone you have just never met:

Who are you?

List 5 interesting things about you

1.

2.

3.

4.

5.

How will you tell them your name in a way that ensures they remember it?

1.

2.

3.

4.

5.

What three other pieces of information will you give?

1.

2.

3.

What is special about you?

Answer: What's special about me is.........

1.

2.

3.

4.

5.

What else is SPECIAL about you?

(List 5 more things. Think about what you are going to get your audience interested in. Things that when your back at work, or playing squash or even on your tea break. They will just have to ask you for more information).

The other thing to watch is if they don't come and ask, your not interesting enough!!

1.

2.

3.

4.

5.

What are you GOOD at ? (List 5 things)

1.

2.

3.

4.

5.

Why is this important to you?

Sometimes in my coaching, I hear people saying "I am not sure if there is anything special about me. I feel like I am just an average Alice/John."

Or, "I would like to think there is something special about me, but I really don't think so…" and you can feel a sense of regret in that tone of voice, almost like the person is trying to say "I wish I could be special, but I have been told I am not, so now I believe it."

Think of it, you've been given talents and abilities in this life for one single purpose: to use them. Yes, all people have talents and abilities. In their own ways. And these special talents and abilities are to be used not only for you, although it all begins with you. These talents and abilities are there to use them – for yourself – but also for all the benefit of all others whose lives you touch.

I know people who happen to shine once for a short time and then disappear in the ocean of statistics that make up our society.

Are you just a statistical number?

In my humble opinion, every person is an individual, with hopes and dreams and desires and plans for the future, and something special about you that makes you … YOU!

Movie quote...

"THERE'S NO CRYING IN BASEBALL"— LEAGUE OF THEIR OWN

"Are you crying? Are you crying? Are you crying?! There's no crying!"

This inspirational speech might not have some deep, insightful message that moves you to your core. But do you really need that when Tom Hanks yells the same phrase in hysterics over and over again? "There's no crying in baseball!" Sometimes we just need a reminder to cut it out with the self-pity. In the middle of a game, or test or interview, you can't just stop and sob. You get it together and get on with it. Thank you for the sound advice right there, Tom.

Stocktaking YOURSELF

How often do you check in on yourself?

How often do you judge how you're doing -- add things up as to where you are in your life and overall happiness.?

A lot!

You do it constantly. Sometimes you're aware of it and other times not.

You look at yourself and ask – Where am I? Who Am I?

It's a deep and important consideration this Who Am I? Because you're taking stock of who you are -- emotionally, physically and spiritually. You're critiquing yourself and holding yourself accountable.

Change is at the heart of it all. The impulse and desire to improve yourself -- to do better and be better.

You think about your health and your age.

You look at your job and make plans to work smarter or drastically change careers so you can do what you love.

Your personal life is also on the block.

All your specific and general thoughts, plans, goals, desires to improve and change are about one thing -- you're looking to be yourself -- to be true to who you really are. True to whom you were born to be.

Add it up...add it up

It's not always easy to find what you want but the answers are in you.

The WHO AM I?

Is a simple addition and subtraction -- including and excluding what you want in and out of your life. You add something to be happier. You take something away for the same reason.

You're organizing your life just as you would organize a desk or cupboard; deciding what is essential and removing what you don't want or need.

Plus and minus are the basics.

Ask for what you want

It's hard to know yourself and figure out exactly what you feel and then what you want.

Start by asking yourself the question and then, find an answer. Follow the thread through to the end. Maybe follow this example:

What do you want?

I want to be happier and much more expressed at work.

Why?

Because I want my life to have meaning and value.

Why?

Because I want to give something to others so people can benefit from my knowledge and skills.

That's what I want.

Taking stock is about finding personal happiness and discovering your life purpose.

Keep asking yourself -- **What do I want?**

Write down whatever comes up until you find the answer at the centre of your heart.

You'll know when you do.

As you begin the process of change, be kind to yourself.

What is missing about you?

1.

2.

3.

How are you not being you?

1.

2.

3.

How do you inhabit yourself?

1.

2.

3.

How are you holding back?

1.

2.

3.

"Stop holding yourself back. If you aren't happy, make a change."
~Unknown

If you're holding yourself back, this may help.

1. Change your attitude to reflect what you want to become.

Your attitude will either move you forward or backwards. It's greatly affected by what you believe, since what you believe determines the decisions you make. Your beliefs largely stem from your past. What people said and did to you and what you concluded those experiences meant about you.

Become aware of what people told you when you were a child and ask yourself if those statements were actually true. Study your accomplishments and your environment, go over what you have done so far and see if they align with the accused statements.

Common answers when people do this exercise:

Untrue fact number one: I am ugly. And yet people outside my family have complimented me on my looks. At first, it was hard for me to believe the compliments were genuine. However, as I observed and listened to the actions and words that followed, I realized that I am not ugly, as my mother led me to believe. We're all beautiful in our own way, and the beauty on the inside is more valuable than what's on the outside.

Untrue fact number two: I was stupid and not good enough, unlike my siblings. And yet I graduated with a degree from a reputable school.

Untrue fact number three: I was useless. And yet the first book called "My Silence Is Broken". Is helping survivors of sexual abuse around the world. And I still have a problem with spelling.

Write yours down and use them to shed any negative beliefs that don't fit into your present situation. You don't necessarily need to get rid of every belief right away, but start with something, no matter how small it may seem, so you can start letting go of your past traumas.

Notes…

2. You know more than you think.

Stop selling yourself short by saying, "I don't know" and instead say, "I will figure it out," and ask yourself "How can I do this better?"

You have the ability to ask for help and connect yourself to the right resources as part of your self-development journey so you can become more, know more, and prepare for the challenges ahead.

The moment I changed my beliefs, I knew that I didn't know everything, but I also knew I had the ability to reach out and get all the tools I needed to complete the work.

3. Let people in.

I started to believe in myself when I decided to surround myself with the right friends and mentors, both from work and at home. I opened up to them about how I felt, what I wanted to improve, and how I wanted to move forward from there.

I believe that having the right people behind you is one of the most critical parts of forming self-belief. That may seem counter-intuitive since self-belief comes from inside, but it's easier to develop confidence when we have people in our lives who believe in us and motivate us to go after the things that will make us happy.

Don't be afraid to reach out to those you feel comfortable with and let them in on what you're going through.

When you believe in yourself enough to reach out to others, trusting that you're worthy of their support, you will become a magnet for opportunities that you never thought were possible

for you. Take a chance, be honest, and life will surprise you.

4. See obstacles as opportunities.

Life will never stop throwing obstacles at you, no matter how

much you try to avoid them. Instead of running from them, learn to see them as opportunities to make what you currently have better.

I used to throw in the towel the moment there was a problem or a glitch in my life and my job. These days, I ask myself, "What are these problems going to teach me? What is life trying to tell me? What are the lessons I'm about to discover?"

Obstacles are there to show you new lessons. The message behind them will only be revealed to those who work hard to overcome them.

What I have learned after successfully completing the project for my new job is that I can do practically anything if I give myself a chance and time to learn and grow. By giving myself a chance in this job, I learned how to approach people better and how to get things done faster, more effectively, and more efficiently.

5. Do not allow defeat to win over triumph.

Remember in the beginning when I said we all have a memory bank? There are two kinds of memory banks. One is "Defeat" and the other is "Triumph." In the first you store all your memories of things you believe you haven't done well; in the second, memories of times when you've succeeded.

Everything you've ever experienced lives in one of these memory banks, which you will withdraw from in the future to inform your decisions. Your choice will inform your habits and behaviour, which ultimately dictate your success and happiness.

Be mindful and guard your mind carefully so you don't allow yourself to withdraw from your "defeat bank account." I didn't, and that was what saved me at the end.

6. Embrace mistakes as teachers.

Don't be too hard on yourself. Mistakes are part of life. I have learned to love them. Though I don't look to make mistakes often, they are my teachers in growth and self-improvement.

During my first job. I was friendly with a few people. We would have lunch together and share our thoughts on the company and our jobs.

Later on, they used the information I shared against me later. Thankfully, I didn't lose my job, but it definitely hurt my chances for future promotions within the company.

Looking back, I'm glad I went through that early in my career, as

it set a strong foundation for how I now interact with colleagues, which helps with my professional achievement. Don't give up just because things get hard.

If you really want something, you have to be prepared to seize opportunities, work hard for it, and never give up.

There were many times during my new job when I wanted to walk over to my boss' office and give my resignation because every

day it was a struggle to get just one thing done. However, deep down I knew that if I quit and went back to my old job, I would live an unhappy, unsatisfying, and regretful life.

Of course, that doesn't mean you should never quit anything. You need to set goals that align with your values. If your values

change along the way, as we all know may happen as we get older, it is okay to give them up and embark on a new journey. Knowing what you really want will help you determine when to

give up and move forward, and when to stick to your guns.

You have the power to overcome the limiting beliefs that stop you from realizing your full potential and creating happiness. It starts with the choice to stop giving them power and start seizing new opportunities.

When I work with Survivors of sexual violence.

I help them understand and help them to change the way they think about their perpetrator. As the more they think about them and hate them, The more powerful the perpetrator becomes. As they are taking up rent-free space in their mind. Don't let them do this.

You are now in control.

Gary Sellors

Author of "My Silence Is Broken"

Your Passion

What matters to you.

What is your passion? (List 3 things, one must not be paid work)

1.

2.

3.

How are you living these passions?

1.

2.

3.

How are they evidenced when you are presenting?

1.

2.

3.

An effective presentation makes the best use of the relationship between the presenter and the audience. It takes full consideration of the audience's needs in order to capture their interest, develop their understanding, inspire their confidence and achieve the presenter's objectives.

Outcomes

Think of a presentation you want to give. With regard to this presentation what do you want for yourself and what do you want for others?

Ask yourself:

What is my outcome for myself?

1.

2.

3.

What is my evidence? What will I see, hear and feel?

Visual (see)

Auditory (hear)

Kinesthetic (feel)

What is my outcome for the others?

What is my evidence? What will I see, hear and feel?

Visual

Auditory

Kinesthetic

States

A state is your way of being at any given moment. It is an indication of the quality of your existence as you interact with the world.

Sequencing states is an art is largely unrecognised. When you are presenting, both you and your audience are moving through different states.

People who are adept at sequencing states are good stand-up comedians, storytellers and inspirational speakers.

Often the audiences are barely aware of the different states they are going through.

Ask yourself:

What state do I want **them** to be in at the beginning?

What state do I want to be in at the beginning?

Them

Myself

What state do I want them to be halfway through?

What state do I want to be in halfway through?

Them

Myself

What state do I want them to be in at the end?

What state do I want to be in at the end?

Them

Myself

Accessing the Positive States

Here are some business frames to put around the process of putting someone into the state:

"As we sit here talking about your business, I'm beginning to wonder if it would be appropriate to ask you now. To recall a time..."

"That reminds me. Can you remember a time when you were totally decisive, now..."

"You know. I was wondering, can you recall a time when you made a business decision that was a big win for you and made you lots of money?"

"And as I ask you so many questions, you may wonder what it would be like to be a client, and as you wonder, if you could just imagine being a client now, you'd probably find that it would be easier to make the right decision..."

"You telling me about your business reminds me of a time when I (pause), well I do wonder if you can recall a time when you totally were satisfied with a purchase you just made."

Metaphors

Storytelling basics:

The characters – you need a hero, plus goodies and baddies along the way

The plot – the storyline of the journey that the hero takes

A conflict – the challenge that the hero takes up or difficulty they face

A resolution – the result or outcome that happens at the end of the tale

Storytelling at work:

Communicate information

Conveys values of the organisation

Educate people

Give the listener the benefit of their wisdom

Help teams to evaluate choices and make decisions

A direct metaphor compares one situation with another where there's an obvious link in terms of the type of content.

An indirect metaphor makes comparisons which are not immediately obvious. Such indirect metaphors form the basis of the most creative advertising campaigns

The main thing is to keep the main thing the main thing.

- Steven Covey

Anchoring

There are five keys to successful anchoring:

1. The first is the intensity of the response or the congruity of the state. In anchoring, we're looking for a fully associated intense state. You may ask, "Are you seeing yourself or are you in your own body?" We want them to be in their own body (associated).

2. The second element is the timing of the anchor. The anchor should be applied just before the peak. If you hold it too long,

then you may find that the person has gone beyond the first experience into a second, into another state, and the two states may be linked.

3. The stimulus should also be unique. The uniqueness of the stimulus is important because if you set up an anchor on an area of the body (assuming a kinesthetic anchor) that is touched a lot, such as a handshake, then the anchor will become weakened

with time (diluted) because it will be set off by other people. So you will want to provide an anchor that is in a unique area of the body.

How long an anchor lasts depends specifically upon how unique the location is. If it's not an intense state that you're anchoring, or

if you haven't stacked it. then the anchor will wear off or dilute itself more quickly. If the location is not unique it can be fired off so many times that it won't work again, because it won't be linked to the specific state.

4. The last key is the replication of the stimulus. The way that you apply the anchor in setting it and in firing it off to test, need to be exactly the same every time. So if you're snapping your fingers or giving them a certain look, you need to do it the same way every time. That anchor needs to be fed back to the person in exactly the same way it was set.

5. The fifth key is the number of times. I.E.: How many times you stacked the anchor.

Circle of Excellence / Confidence Building

Do this exercise:

Picture a circle in front of you on the floor

Think of a resource that you want, and remember a time when you had it.

Now step in the circle and re-live that experience (make it real), anchor.

Step back out

Repeat with another resource and relive the experience.

Step back in (repeat 3 times total) anchor.

Think of a coming event, press anchor as you step into the circle.

You are ready to go

The answer (where butterflies equate to fear) is clear and simple in the following maxim:

To calm the butterflies you must be relaxed. To be relaxed you must be confident. To be confident you must be prepared and rehearsed.

Good preparation is the key to confidence, which is the key to being relaxed, and this calms the butterflies,(i.e., overcomes the fear).

Movie quote...

"Our deepest fear is that we are powerful beyond measure. It is our light, not our darkness, that most frightens us." - Get Carter

The first few words of this speech should sound familiar. They were borrowed from a poem written by Marianne Williamson

titled "Our Deepest Fear." Perhaps our we don't fear inadequacy. Have you ever even considered that, deep down, you really fear

to reach the full potential of your power? Maybe we really do set ourselves up to "play small." We should not be ashamed of confidence.

Spatial Anchoring

Spatial anchoring is a way of influencing your audience through anchors.

When you repeatedly do the same thing on stage in the same place, then people come to expect certain behaviour from you according to where you move around the stage.

A lectern is a definite anchor – when you stand at the lectern, people expect you to speak.

Defeat is not defeated unless

accepted as a reality-in your own

mind.

- Bruce Lee

Body Movement / Walking Patterns

Changing your position or location while speaking is the broadest, most visible physical action you can perform.

Therefore it can either help drive your message home or spell failure for even the most well-planned speech.

Moving your body in a controlled, purposeful manner creates three benefits:

1. Supports and reinforces what you say

2. Attracts an audience's attention

3. Burns up nervous energy and relieves physical tension

However, body movement can work against you. Remember this one rule:

NEVER MOVE WITHOUT A REASON

The eye is inevitably attracted to a moving object, so anybody movement you make during a speech invites attention. Too much movement, even the right kind, can become distracting to an audience.

Bear in mind the following types of body movement:

Stepping forward during a speech suggest you are arriving at an important point.

Stepping backwards indicates you've concluded an idea and want the audience to relax for a moment.

Lateral movement implies a transitional it indicates that you are leaving one thought and taking up another. For example, if you are ready to move on to your next point, move slowly sideways until you are standing next to the lectern.

The final reason for body movement is the easiest; to get from one place to another. In almost every speaking situation, you must walk from the location you are addressing your audience to your props, especially if you are using visual aids.

Always change positions by leading with the foot nearest your destination.

You may ask, why move in the first place?

Moving forces people to focus and follow you. The way you walk from your seat to the speaker's location is very important. When you are introduced, you should appear eager to speak.

Many speakers look as though they are heading towards execution.

Walk confidently from your seat to the lectern. Pause there a few seconds and then move out from behind the lectern. It is wise to use the lectern as a point of departure, not a barrier to hide behind.

Smile before you say your first words.

Don't stand too close or move beyond the first row of people.

Walking stresses an important idea. It is essential that you walk with purpose and intention, not just a random shift of position.

For example, taking about three steps, moving at a slight angle, usually works best.

Use three positions with visual aids, your "home" position is front and centre. The other two positions should be relatively near the "home" position.

You can move to the right of the lectern and then to the left.

Using and varying these three positions prevents you from favouring one side of the audience. If you're speaking on stage, these three positions are called front centre, stage left, and stage right.

Never stand in front of any visual aid.

Practice your walking patterns to and from your three positions. These positions should be planned just as your hand gestures are, to some degree.

For example, you want your body to move and gesture naturally.

However, since most people are nervous about speaking in public, they tend to stiffen their muscles and hold back their natural tendency to gesture. Let your body tell you when it wants to move.

"Words are not visuals,

They are for listening to"

What's your favourite sense?

Pick A – B – C on these questions

If only three rooms are left at a beach resort, I'll choose the room that offers?

A) An ocean view but lots of noise.

B) Sounds of the ocean but no view.

C) Comfort but lots of noise and no view.

When I have a problem?

A) I look for alternatives.

B) I talk about the problem.

C) I rearrange the details.

When riding in a car, I want the inside too?

A) Look good.

B) Sound quiet or powerful.

C) Feel comfortable or secure.

When I explain a concert or event I've just attended, I first?

A) Describe how it looked.

B) Tell people how it sounded.

C) Convey the feeling.

In my spare time, I most enjoy?

A) Watching TV or going to the movies.

B) Reading or listening to music.

C) Doing something physical.

The one thing I personally believe everyone should experience in his or her lifetime is?

A) Sight.

B) Sound

C) Feeling.

Of the following activities, I spend the most time indulging in?

A) Daydreaming.

B) Listening to my thoughts.

C) Picking up on my feelings.

When someone is trying to convince me of something?

A) I want to see evidence or proof.

B) I talk myself through it.

C) I trust my intuition.

I usually speak and think?

A) Quickly.

B) Moderately.

C) Slowly.

Do I breathe from?

A) High in my chest.

B) Low in my chest.

C) My belly.

When finding my way around an unfamiliar city?

A) I use a map.

B) I ask for directions.

C) I trust my Intuition.

When I choose clothes, it is important to me that?

A) I look immaculate.

B) I make a personal statement about my personality.

C) I feel comfortable.

When I chose a restaurant, my main concern is that?

A) It looks impressive.

B) I can hear myself talk.

C) I will be comfortable.

Do I make decisions?

A) Quickly.

B) Moderately.

C) Slowly.

Your Score:-

A 's =   Visual.

B 's =   Auditory.

C 's =   Kinesthetic.

Favoured Representation Systems

V: Visual

People who are visual often stand or sit with their heads and/or bodies erect, with their eyes up. They will be breathing from the top of their lungs. They often sit forward in their chair and tend to be organized, neat, well-groomed and orderly.

They are often thin and wiry. They memorize by seeing pictures and are less distracted by noise. They often have trouble remembering verbal instructions because their minds tend to wander.

A visual person will be interested in how your program LOOKS. Appearances are important to them.

A: Auditory

People who are auditory will quite often move their eyes sideways. They breathe from the middle of their chest. They typically talk to themselves and can be easily distracted by noise. (Some even move their lips when they talk to themselves.)

They can repeat things back to you easily, they learn by listening, and usually like music and talking on the phone.

They memorize by steps, procedures, and sequences (sequentially).

The auditory person likes to be TOLD how they're doing and responds to a certain tone of voice or set of words. They will be interested in what you have to say about your program.

K: Kinesthetic

People who are kinesthetic will typically be breathing from the bottom of their lungs, so you will see their stomach go in and out when they breathe. They often move and talk verrry slowly.

They respond to physical rewards and touching. They also stand closer to people than a visual person. They memorize by doing or walking through something. They will be interested in your program if it "feels right", or if you can give them something they can grasp.

Ai: Auditory Digital

This person will spend a fair amount of time talking to themselves. They will want to know if your program "makes sense".

The auditory digital person can exhibit characteristics of the other major representational systems.

List of predicate phrases

VISUAL

An eyeful

Appears to me

Beyond a shadow of a   doubt

Bird's eye view

Catch a glimpse of

Clear cut

Dim view

Flashed on

 Get a perspective on

Get a scope on

Hazy Idea

House of a different colour

In light of

In person

In view of

Looks like

Make a scene

Mental image

Mental picture

Mind's eye

Naked eye

Paint a picture

See to it

Short-sighted

Showing off

Sight for sore eyes

Staring off into space

Take a peek

Tunnel vision

Well defined

AUDITORY

Afterthought

Blabbermouth

Clear as a bell

Clearly expressed

Gallon

Describe in detail

Earful

Give an account of

Give me your ear

Grant an audience

Heard voices

Hidden message

Hold your tongue

Idle talk

Inquire into

Keynote speaker

Loud and clear

Manner of speaking

Pay attention to

Power of speech

Purrs like a kitten

State your purpose

Tattle-tale

To tell the truth

Tongue-tied

Tuned in/tuned out

Unheard of

Utterly

Voiced an opinion

Well informed

Within hearing

Word for word

KINESTHETIC

All washed up

Boils down to

Chip off the old block

Come to grips with

Control yourself

Cool/calm/collected

Firm foundations

Get a handle on

Get a load of this

Get in touch with

Get the drift of

Get your goat

Hand in hand

Hang in there

Heated argument

Hold it!

Hold on!

Hothead

Keep your shirt on

Know-how

Lay cards on the table

Pain-in-the-neck

Pull some strings

Sharp as a tack

Slipped my mind

Smooth operator

So Tough

Start from scratch

Stiff upper lip

Stuffed shirt

Too much of a hassle

Topsy-turvy

If this LOOKS GOOD, to you we will go ahead and FOCUS on getting the paperwork in.

If this SOUNDS GOOD, to you we will go ahead and DISCUSS how to set up an account.

If this FEELS GOOD, to you we will go ahead & set up an account by HANDLING THE PAPERWORK.

Your future – created by – what you do TODAY – not tomorrow

Movie quote...

"Well, you want to know what I see? I see pride!

I see power! I see a bad-a** mother who doesn't take no

crap off nobody!" "PRIDE"—COOL RUNNINGS

We all get down on ourselves sometimes. Your perceived

social standing do not define you. You are special. You are

awesome. This scene shows you how to own that, and if it requires

some shouting in a mirror to get the message across, then hey, I

say go for it.

Top 4 Ways To Let Yourself Be Heard

Do people often tell you that they can't hear you or understand what you're saying?

You may think it's because you are not speaking loudly enough. But actually, the volume may be only part of the problem.

I suggest doing a systems check on these four areas:

Articulation / Pronunciation

Vocal Volume Level

Voice Projection

The Way You Feel About Yourself

1. Articulation / Pronunciation

There is a difference between not being heard (being inaudible) and not being understood (being unintelligible). Sometimes

people confuse the two. Unintelligibility may be caused by problems with articulation and pronunciation.

People with poor articulation can sound throaty because their tongue is pulled too far back, or they may sound muffled

because they don't move their tongue enough when they speak. Both problems affect our ability to be understood.

Make sure your tongue is positioned toward the front of your mouth and that you use your tongue to clearly enunciate your words.

If you mispronounce your words you will also have a difficult

time being understood.

Brush up on pronunciation skills by consulting a good

pronouncing dictionary.

2. Controlling Vocal Volume

Imagine that your voice has a volume knob with five settings:

1-WHISPER

2-SOFT

3-CONVERSATIONAL

4-LOUD

5-SHOUT

For normal and healthy conversational speech, do not use volume levels 1 or 5. Both can strain the voice. Shout only in an emergency and save your whispers for the library, theatre or bedroom.

Strive to speak most of the time at volume level 3. Use levels 2 and 3 for colour, emphasis and variety. A conversational level will differ with each situation.

To be heard it must be adjusted so that we are speaking at a level that is slightly louder than the background noise around us. Obviously, there is much more background noise, for example, in a crowded restaurant than in a quiet conference room.

3. Projecting Your Voice

Volume level should not be confused with projection. To project the voice, don't try to yell or force it out of your body. This causes strain. To have a voice that carries well, you must use your body's natural resonators.

Your body has three resonating cavities: the voice box, the mouth and the nose. The voice is produced at the vocal cords and then amplified in the facial mask around the lips and nose.

Speech therapist of mine says the simplest way to find your facial mask is to hum. Try it now. HMMMMMMMM. Good.

Now practice alternating humming and speaking. HMMMMM My name is Susan. HMMMMMy favourite colour is blue.

HMMMMany people say I'm a great dancer... etc. Have fun with it.

Practice humming and speaking throughout the day. Once you get the hang of what a resonant voice feels like, you can drop the hum and feel the vibration of your words in your facial mask.

4.   The Way You Feel About Yourself

It is found that there is often a strong psychological component to communication difficulties. Soft speakers may unconsciously be trying to hold themselves back, inhibit their self-expression, or stifle themselves, and these factors should be explored.

Eye Pattern chart

IMAGINED VISUAL

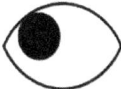 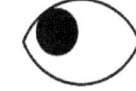

Up and to the right

- creating a picture of something never seen
- creative visualization
- possibly lying or making up a visual

VISUAL MEMORY

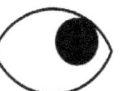 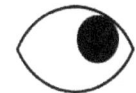

Up and to the left

- remembering a picture or image
- recalling a scene witnessed

IMAGINED AUDITORY

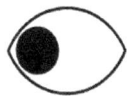 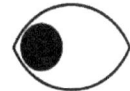

To the right

- imagine one sound morphing into another
- making up a tune
- writing a poem
- possibly lying or making up words

AUDITORY MEMORY

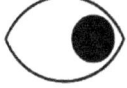 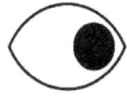

To the left

- remembering a sound
- recalling a tune previously heard
- remembering a poem

FEELINGS

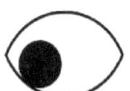 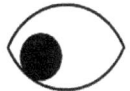

Down and to the right

- recalling an emotion
- imagining an emotion
- remembering a physical feeling
- imagining a physical feeling

INTERNAL SELF TALK

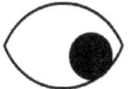 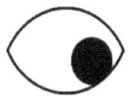

Down and to the left

- listening to the voice inside
- talking to oneself

Right Up - Visual Constructed

Left Up - Visual Remembered

Right Middle - Auditory Constructed

Left Middle - Auditory Remembered

Right Down- Auditory Digital (Self-talk)

Left Down - Kinesthetic (Feelings)

Representational System Questions

Visual Remembered – Left Up

In your immediate family, whose eyes are the darkest?

Name four things that were on your desk last time you saw it?

How many pictures are in the hall outside this room?

What kind of flowers did you last give/receive?

What colour were the walls in your first bedroom?

Who were the first 5 people you saw today?

Visual Constructed – Right Up

What colour would you like your next car to be?

What would I look like with purple hair?

How much is 367 plus 48?

Imagine seeing yourself sitting here from a position 3 feet behind yourself

How would you look in a clown's costume?

Auditory Remembered – Left Middle

What was the last excuse you told someone?

Listen to the first few notes of Beethoven's 5th Symphony

What is the difference between a police siren and an ambulance?

Whose voice do you have most difficulty understanding on the telephone?

When walking, which pair of shoes makes the most noise?

Auditory Construct – Right Middle

What would your voice sound like if you had Donald duck's voice?

Kinesthetic – Right Down

Which is warmer - your right or your left hand?

When was the last time you overate?

What is one of your happiest memories?

Describe the feeling of your favourite article of clothing

How to Use Transitions Effectively

Transitions are an integral part of a smooth flowing presentation, yet many speakers forget to plan their transitions. The primary purpose of a transition is to lead your listener from one idea to another.

The following are some examples of transitions that work well:

Bridge words or phrases

(Furthermore, meanwhile, however, in addition, consequently, finally.

Trigger transition (same word or idea used twice:

"A similar example is ...").

Ask a Question ("How many of you ....?")

Flashback ("Do you remember when I said ...?")

Point-By-Point ("There are three points ...The first one is.. The second one is..etc.)

Add a Visual Aid as a Transition

Many times it may be appropriate to add a visual between your regular visual aids for the sole purpose of a "visual" transition.

Many times a clever cartoon used here can add some humour to your presentations.

Pausing. Even a simple pause, when effectively used, can act as a transition. This allows the audience to "think" about what was just said and give it more time to register.

Use Physical Movement. The speaker should move or change the location of their body. This is best done when you are changing to a new idea or thought.

Use a Personal Story The use of a story, especially a personal one is a very effective technique used by many professional speakers. Used effectively, it can help reinforce any points you made during your presentation.

Use the PEP formula (Point, Example, Point) (This is a very common format used and can also be combined with the use of a personal story. Make sure stories or examples you use help reinforce your message.

Three common mistakes made when using transitions:

1. The most common mistake people make is that they DON'T use transitions at all. Transitions help your information flow from one idea to the next.

2. The second most common mistake is using transitions that are too short. Not enough time is spent bridging to the next idea. This is extremely important when changing to a new section of ideas within your presentation.

3. The third most common mistake is that people use the same transition throughout the presentation. This becomes very boring after a short while. Try to be creative with your transitions.

Transitions and the Team Presentation

Transitions become extremely important when a team presentation is involved. The transition from one speaker to the next must be planned and skilfully executed. Each speaker

should use a brief introduction of the next topic and speaker as part of this transition.

Rapport

Desired Outcome:

To be able to establish rapport with any person, at any moment in time.

Theory:

A.   Communication is:

7%   WORDS

38% TONALITY

55% PHYSIOLOGY

B.   When people are like each other, they like each other.

Rapport is a process of responsiveness, not necessarily "liking".

Process:

A.   Rapport is established by matching & mirroring

Matching and Mirroring

Rapport

Matching

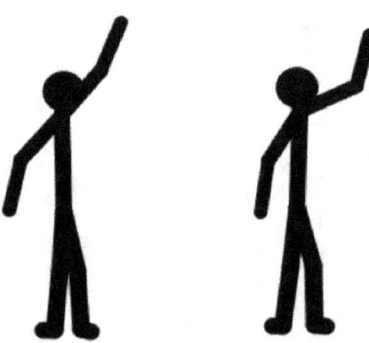

Rapport

Mirroring

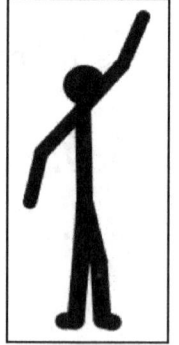 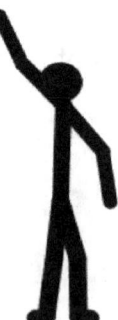

B. The major elements of rapport: (Key elements marked with " * ")

PHYSIOLOGY   (55%)

Posture *

Gesture

Facial expression & blinking *

Breathing

TONALITY   (38%)

Voice

Tone   (pitch)

Tempo   (speed)

Timbre   (quality)

Volume   (loudness)

WORDS   (7%)

Predicates

Keywords

Common experiences & associations

Content chunks

EXERCISE:

Do a presentation, while mirroring people in the audience

"You Don't Need

To Waste Your

Time On Someone

Who Only Wants

You Around

When It Fits

Their Needs"

Elements of an Effective Speech

"Half the world is composed of people who have something to say and can't; The other half have nothing to say and keep saying it."

Anyone can give a speech. Not everyone can give an effective speech. To give an effective speech there are 6 elements you should consider.

Be Prepared - Being prepared is by far the most important element.

How many times do you practice your speech? As a general rule, you should spend about 30 hours of preparation and rehearsal time for every hour you will be speaking.

Use a tape recorder or videotape yourself. This will help you to get an accurate picture of how you speak.

Give of Yourself - Use personal examples and stories in your speech whenever possible. Make sure your stories help to emphasise or support your point. The stories must match your message. Use examples from your personal and professional

life to making your point. In either case be willing to give part of yourself by sharing some of yourself with the audience.

Stay Relaxed - To stay relaxed you should be prepared. Also, focus on your message and not the audience. Use gestures, including walking patterns. Practice the opening of your speech and plan exactly how you will say it. The audience will judge you

in the first 30 seconds they see you.

Use Natural Humour - Don't try to be a stand-up comedian. Use natural humour by poking fun at yourself and something you said or did. Be sure NOT to make fun of anyone in the audience.

People will laugh with you when you poke fun at yourself but don't overdo it.

Plan Your Body & Hand Positions - During the practice of your speech look for occasions where you can use a gesture.

Establish three positions where you will stand and practice not only how to move to them but where in your speech do you move.

Pick three positions, one on centre stage, one to your right, and one to your left. Do not hide behind the lectern.

When you do move. Maintain eye contact with the audience.

Pay attention to all details - Make sure you have the right location (school, hotel, room & time). Make sure you know how to get to where you are speaking.

Ask how large an audience you will be speaking to. Make sure you bring all your visual aids and plenty of handouts.

Arrive early so you can check out where you will be speaking and make any last minute adjustments.

It is very important that you pay attention to even the smallest details.

You can never over plan.

Remember,

"He who fails to plan is planning

for failure"

The 'Yes but...' Game (Fun)

Get your friends in a circle

Person A begins with (round one) with offering 'a good idea'

Person B replies 'Yes, but...' and offers their own idea.

Person C and all the other team members offer their ideas in turn, always starting with 'Yes, but...'

A thought:-

When we are participants at a presentation, we are like pedestrians who criticise road hogs- we complain about boring, long-winded speeches.

Then, like drivers who ignore pedestrians, we get up to make our presentation and do exactly the same

"The world hasn't changed – you have just got a better understanding of what is going on"

Preparing your presentation

The 3 W's – Why – What -Who

Why?

Why am I going to give this presentation?

To provide information

To represent the company

To entertain

To fill up the agenda

To sell my ideas

To defend my position

Whatever the answer, keep asking "why" in other ways …..

What is the objective I wish to achieve

What is happening now that I wish to change or clarify

What will I accept as evidence that my speech has succeeded

What must the audience do or think at the end

…… until it becomes obvious what your essential messages must be.

What?

Answering the question "why?" properly will tell you what your main messages should be but, however intelligent your

audience, they will neither want nor be able to absorb more

than :

4 or 5 Key points

Since you have a lot of competition from other speakers you need a vehicle to carry your message to the audience; after all, if your presentation is not memorable – why bother to speak?

A mnemonic device to link key messages together and help retention i.e. …

A series of slides to package your messages

An example to make a bridge between your messages and the audience's experience

Who?

Once you know exactly why you are going to make the presentation and what your key points will be, you must ask, who will be in the audience?

So as to customise your message and make it stick.

Who are the participants? Level? Background?

What do they already know about the subject?

Are they really interested? (If not, you have to create the interest)

How fast can they absorb what I'm saying?

What do they expect me to say?

What is their mindset (prejudices, attitudes, beliefs, etc)

To be safe and have your speech tailored to the audience, play devils advocate and ask, 'How could I best offend them if I really wanted to ?'

Peripheral vision

Using your peripheral vision – opening out your visual field to its very edges – is a helpful tool to feel more relaxed, open and 'spacious' in front of a group (or indeed whenever you want to feel that way).

Why you need to practise

It's important to practice expanding our visual field because it's not an obvious response when we're speaking to groups! In fact, we do the opposite, which is probably to do with our deep-wired connections between distance and safety around an external stressor. When we're agitated, our field of vision decreases – we become tunnel-visioned – in order to deal with the threat. We tend to look down, too.

What then happens is that we 'focus in' even more on our discomfort. This also has the detrimental effect of decreasing eye-contact with our audience, especially people at the outer sides of the group.

Test it out now

Try expanding your vision field now: start to become aware of what's in the outer reach of your vision; soften your eyes and, if you like, hold your hand in front of your face and gradually move

it to the side until you can barely see it anymore. You can

probably go further than you think!

How this helps

Deliberately using your peripheral vision is another way of changing your focus, mentally as well as physically.

This can help your speaking in 3 ways:

You feel calmer because your sense of personal space expands; you feel less hemmed in and pressured

You become more externally aware of the room and of your audience (this is a good thing, promise! Keep reading to get more information on why it helps)

These 2 things result in the audience feeling more connected to you.

A connecting loop forms between speaker and audience – which is what we're after.

Movie quote...

 "How you play today, from this moment on, is how you will be remembered. This is your opportunity to rise from these ashes and grab the glory. We are…Marshall!"

 "WE ARE MARSHALL"

Ah, another tear-jerker, but nonetheless an inspiring speech by Matthew McConaughey's character, Jack Lengyel. "The Thundering Herd show that even through adversity and times of struggle, a community can come together through football."

Setting it up

People speak very differently depending on their audience. You might tell your friend's things that you would never share with your families and you use very different language with your colleagues than you do at home.

This filtering or catering to different audiences is something you do naturally, without even thinking about it. However, you're less likely to apply the same logic when speaking in front of a group.

Why?

Because one of the most frightening things about public speaking is that you're standing up in front of a room full of strangers. It's very hard to know the right thing to say at a networking event when faced with small groups of three or four people you've never met. Selecting the best topic, theme, or content for 20, 200, or 500 people is even harder.

The trick is getting to know your audience. In fact, it's the number one thing you should do before you agree to headline an event, choose a topic or embark on your research.

You're probably thinking: This is crazy advice. I don't have time to get to know 200 people! You're right, you don't. And you don't need to know them in a what they had for breakfast kind of way. You do need to know why they're at the event and what they want to hear.

Here are five questions to ask to help you get to know your audience before you walk in the room.

1. What Kind of People Will Be in the Room?

If the event organizer doesn't know who'll be there, ask for the attendee list. If it doesn't exist yet, ask for the list from the previous year's event. You'll be able to see from the job titles and companies what the level and industry of the audience is.

Ask yourself: Are these the kinds of people I should be speaking to? Are they potential clients or customers? Are they potential investors? If the answer to all of these questions is "no," think carefully about why you're agreeing to the event. Preparing a presentation or a speech takes a long time, and delivering it takes huge emotional energy. Only expend time and energy on public speaking gigs that deliver your message to your target audience.

2. What's the Theme of the Event or Conference?

Make sure you know what the theme is and how your presentation connects with it. This sounds like an obvious one, but all too often it's a question that's forgotten. If everyone's turning up to hear about innovation and you want to talk about customer service, this is probably the wrong event for you.

However, if you can find a way to talk about innovation in customer service, you could be onto a winner. The theme tells you why people are going to the event. So, naturally, the audience will be more interested in what you have to say if you give them new insights on the topic they've signed up to learn about.

3. What Are They Most Afraid Of?

This sounds like a strange question to ask an event organizer, but it's a really important one. At different times, it's likely you'll find yourself speaking to people from different industries, professions, or at very different stages in their career—and your approach should vary accordingly.

For example, if you're a go-to tech expert, it might be that in many rooms, everyone nods when you discuss upcoming trends. But what about an audience that's new to the game? If they're afraid that they're already behind the curve, you'll isolate them by diving in headfirst. But, if you know their fears, you can include additional context and explanation, making them feel comfortable and delivering a more impactful speech.

4. What Are They Excited About?

Now that you know who's in the room and what they might be afraid of, try and find out what gets them excited. If it's an

industry that you're less familiar with, ask the event organizer or an industry expert if there are any big trends to be aware of.

As you may know, storytelling is a big trend in speechwriting and presentations at the moment—and it's one I personally use to generate excitement. Another insider tip is discussing the latest thing. Try to give your audience some new insight to take back to the office and share with their colleagues. (Bonus: It will also position you as a thought leader who's ahead of the curve.)

5. Whom Do You Respond To?

Don't forget to learn from your own experience as an audience member! If someone hooked you with a great story, think about which of your experiences you could use in a similar way. If someone bored you to tears with a presentation of 60 slides, keep your slides to no more than 10.

If you need inspiration, watch some TED talks or speeches online. You'll soon learn what you like, what you don't, and why.

https:www.ted.com/talks

Copy what you like and ditch the rest: It will help you develop your own unique style as a speaker.

Getting to know your audience is critical for public speaking success. It will help you make better decisions about which gigs to agree to and which to sidestep. It will help you to find the right content for the room, and it will act as a guide for how to present it.

And with these five questions, you can get to know the audience without ever even meeting them.

Think of something you don't like – attracts more negative thinking

Your mind is very powerful. Yet, if you're like most people, you probably spend very little time reflecting on the way you think. After all, who thinks about thinking?

But, the way you think about yourself turns into your reality. If you draw inaccurate conclusions about who you are and what you're capable of doing, you'll limit your potential.

The Link between Thoughts, Feelings And Behaviour

Your thoughts are a catalyst for self-perpetuating cycles. What you think directly influences how you feel and how you behave. So if you think you're a failure, you'll feel like a failure. Then, you'll act like a failure, which reinforces your belief that you must be a failure.

I see this happen all the time in my therapy office. Someone will come in saying, "I'm just not good enough to advance in my career." That assumption leads her to feel discouraged and causes her to put in less effort. That lack of effort prevents her from getting a promotion.

Or, someone will say, "I'm really socially awkward." So when that individual goes to a social gathering, he stays to in the corner by himself. When no one speaks to him, it reinforces his belief that he must be socially awkward.

Your negative thinking gets reinforced

Once you draw a conclusion about yourself, you're likely to do two things; look for evidence that reinforces your belief and discount anything that runs contrary to your belief.

Someone who develops the belief that he's a failure, for example, will view each mistake as proof that he's not good enough. When he does succeed at something, he'll chalk it up to luck.

Consider for a minute that it might not be your lack of talent or lack of skills that are holding you back. Instead, it might be your beliefs that keep you from performing at your peak.

Creating a more positive outlook can lead to better outcomes. That's not to say positive thoughts have magical powers. But optimistic thoughts lead to productive behaviour, which increases your chances of a successful outcome.

Challenge Your Thinking

Take a look at the labels you've placed on yourself. Maybe you've declared yourself incompetent. Or perhaps you've decided you're a bad leader.

Remind yourself that you don't have to allow those beliefs to restrict your potential. Just because you think something, doesn't make it true.

The good news is, you can change how you think. You can alter your perception and change your life. Here are two ways to challenge your beliefs:

Look for evidence to the contrary. Take note of any times when your beliefs weren't reinforced. Acknowledging exceptions to the rule will remind you that your belief isn't always true.

Challenge your beliefs. Perform behavioural experiments that test how true your beliefs really are. If you think you're not good enough, do something that helps you to feel worthy. If you've labelled yourself too wimpy to step outside of your comfort zone, force yourself to do something that feels a little uncomfortable.

With practice, you can train your brain to think differently. When you give up those self-limiting beliefs, you'll be better equipped to reach your greatest potential.

EXERCISE: (Balls) fun

With peripheral vision

Do 7 minutes presentation with distractions - people throwing plastic balls at you from different angles in the crowd, as a distraction. You catch them and return them. Just one ball at a time.

It's a fun exercise and shows you how it is to keep focused on your presentation with so many distractions in your peripheral vision. Most people will give up before 7 minutes. Enjoy, its fun and a silly game.

MIND MAPS

Mind Mapping is a process that involves a distinct combination of imagery, colour and visual-spatial arrangement. The technique maps out your thoughts using keywords that trigger associations in the brain to spark further ideas.

Mind mapping is simply a diagram used to visually represent or outline information. It is a powerful graphic technique you can use to translate what's in your mind into a visual picture. Since mind mapping works like the brain does it allows you to organize and understand information faster and better?

Mind mapping is one of the best ways to capture your thoughts and bring them to life in visual form. Beyond just note-taking, though, mind maps can help you become more creative, remember more, and solve problems more effectively. Whether you're new to mind maps or just want a refresher, here's all you need to know about this technique.

A mind map is basically a diagram that connects information around a central subject. I like to think of it as a tree, although it has more of a radial structure. In any case, at the centre is your main idea, say, poetry, and the branches are subtopics or related ideas, such as types of poetry, famous poets, and poetry publications. Greater levels of detail branch out from there and branches can be linked together.

Mind maps can be used for pretty much any thinking or learning task, from studying a subject (such as a new language) to planning your career or even building better habits. They're great for teams to use as well, for group brainstorming and interactive presentations.

How to do your Mind Map

Start in the CENTRE of a blank page turned sideways. Why? Because starting in the centre gives your Brain freedom to spread out in all directions and to express itself more freely and naturally.

Use an IMAGE or PICTURE for your central idea. Why? Because an image is worth a thousand words and helps you use your Imagination. A central image is more interesting, keeps you focused, helps you concentrate, and gives your Brain more of a buzz!

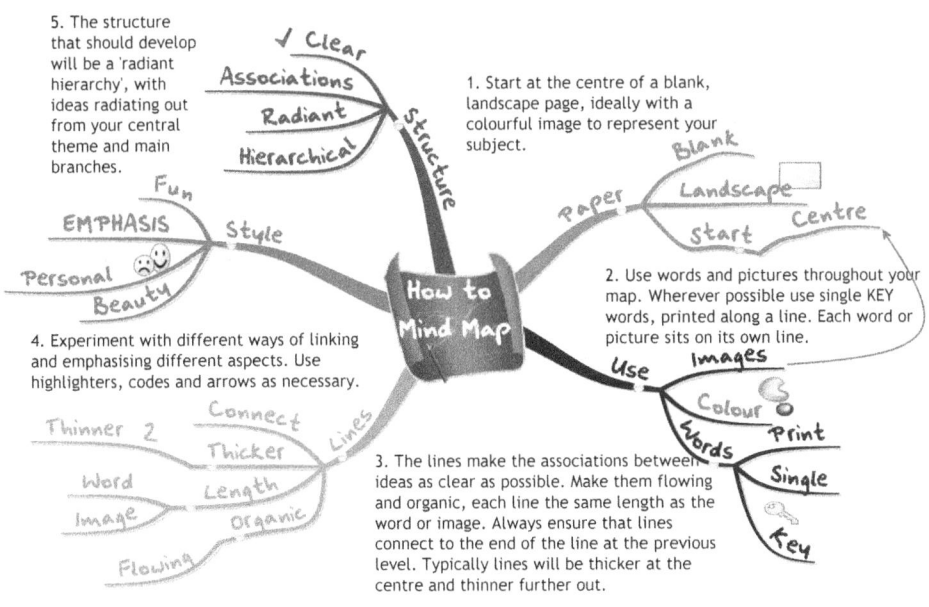

Use COLOURS throughout. Why? Because colours are as exciting to your Brain as are images. Colour adds extra vibrancy and life to your Mind Map, adds tremendous energy to your Creative Thinking, and is fun!

CONNECT your MAIN BRANCHES to the central image and connect your second- and third-level branches to the first and second levels, etc. Why? Because your brain works by association. It likes to link two (or three, or four) things together. If you connect the branches, you will understand and remember a lot more easily.

Make your branches CURVED rather than straight-lined. Why? Because having nothing but straight lines are boring to your Brain.

Use ONE KEYWORD PER LINE. Why Because single keywords give your Mind Map more power and flexibility.

Use IMAGES throughout. Why because each image, like the central image, is also worth a thousand words. So if you have only 10 images in your Mind Map, it's already the equal of 10,000 words of notes!

For further information and inspiration, check out these mind map galleries and other resources, which illustrate the many ways you can use mind maps in your life:

- Mappio - mind map gallery

- Mind Map Art - gallery of beautiful hand-drawn mind maps

- MindMappingStrategies - a blog about mind mapping

- Mind-Mapping.org - one of the most extensive resources about mind mapping software

- Learning Fundamentals - tricks of the trade for mind mapping, particularly on paper

4 Common Ways to Remember Material

Remembering speeches can be a very intimidating experience.

There are many ways one can remember the material.

Memorising

Reading from complete text

Using Notes

Using Visual Aids as Notes

Memorising.

This is can be absolutely the worst way to keep track of material. People are preoccupied with trying to remember the words to say and not the ideas behind the words (or with the audience).

As a result, normal voice inflexion disappears. With memorising, mental blocks become inevitable. With memorising it is not a matter of "will" you forget; it's a matter of WHEN!

Reading from complete text.

Listening to someone read a speech or presentation is hated by most people. People say, "If that's all they were going to do is read their speech, I could have read it myself."

I'm sure many of us have experienced this at least once while attending a conference or two.

Below are some reasons why I believe people read poorly:

The speaker loses normal voice inflexion because they lose touch with the ideas behind the words.

Listen for pauses. Natural speech is filled with pauses; unnatural speech is not.

The text hasn't spoken the language - too often speakers write their speeches in "business language". That is often hard to read, much less listened to.

The speech isn't static - the potted plant will probably move more.

There is little movement, little energy, and little interest behind the lectern.

There's no or little eye contact - any eye contact is with the text, not the audience.

To read the text while trying to maintain eye contact with the audience takes a lot of practice.

The speaker is scared - many speakers read because they are afraid to try anything else. They know reading will fail but at least it will fail with a small "f" rather than a capital one.

NOTE: There are times when speeches MUST be read. Many times it is necessary to read policy statements or company announcements.

Also, some speeches must be timed right down to the second. When you have to read!

If reading is absolutely necessary, here are some suggestions:

Pay attention to the inflexion in your voice - to sound natural, rehearse often, checking yourself for pauses. Ask yourself if your words sound the way you would say them if you weren't reading. Tape yourself and listen to your own voice.

Take notes where changes should be made with the inflexion in your voice.

When preparing your written speech, say the words "out loud" first in order that your written text will read closer to your speaking style. This will make it easier to read and much easier to listen to.

People often DO NOT write the same way as they speak and this makes reading more difficult. If we use wording and phrasing we normally use in our everyday language it will be easier to add the correct voice inflexion and tone.

Annotate your text to indicate which words to emphasise. Numbers are the easiest target words to say slowly with emphasis on each syllable.

One of the biggest problems speakers' face when reading text is that we often forget to use gestures. We are so busy making sure we read the text we fail to communicate effectively with our entire body.

One thing we can do to help this is to "double space" your typed text to leave room to add notes or cues about gestures and other reminder type clues.

We need to practice using this annotated text of our speech so we can easily and smoothly react to these cues for our gestures while at the same time correctly read the text. This does take some practice. Some people do this very effectively.

Record yourself reading the speech and then sit and watch the speech, making notes as to the gestures, which could have been used.

Add notes to your written text based on this review, using notes or even pictures of the gestures to use and deliver the speech again, trying this time to add gestures. After a little practice, this will become second nature.

When we read speeches, the amount of eye contact with our audience is usually less. In some cases, people who read speeches have NO eye contact.

To avoid this, first, write as you speak. When typing the text, use upper and lower case letters.

This will make it easier to read. <TYPING EVERYTHING IN UPPER CASE, AS I HAVE DONE HERE, MAKES IT MORE DIFFICULT TO READ>

Don't have long paragraphs or you will lose your place every time you look up. Start a new paragraph every sentence or two. Also, have your text double-spaced. Some people even go so far as alternating the colour of the text for each paragraph.

Use unstapled pages for your text. Paperclip your pages and just before you begin, remove the paper clip. As you prepare your text, keep in mind that you will have to handle these pages and you want to do this smoothly and as quietly as you can.

Do not have part of a sentence begin on one page and continue onto the next page. End the page with a complete sentence and paragraph.

During your pauses, smoothly "slide" the page you just finished using to one side and continue with the text on the next page. Do not pick up the page and place it behind or turn the page over when done. This will be distracting and will bring attention to the fact that you are reading. Avoid handling the pages as much as possible while you are reading.

With a lot of practice and careful preparation, you can deliver a powerful speech, even when reading. Some of the world's greatest speeches were read, but you can be assured, they weren't reading them for the first time when delivering their speech to their audience.

Practice, practice, practice.

Using Notes

This is the most common way for remembering the material. Using notes is better than reading since the speaker can have normal voice inflexion and make more effective eye contact.

If your notes are on the lectern, you probably won't move very far from them. If notes are in your hand, you probably won't gesture very much.

Below are some suggestions to consider if you decide to use notes:

USING NOTES

Use note cards. Include quotes, statistics and lists you may need, NOT paragraphs of text. VERY IMPORTANT: Number your note cards! (Just in case you drop them).

Don't put too much information on each note card or you will find yourself reading too much. Put only a few words or key phrases.

Leave your notes on the lectern or table and move away occasionally. Don't be afraid to move away from your notes and get out of your comfort zone. Too many speakers use the lectern to hide behind and this restricts the effective use of your entire body.

Practice using your note cards. If you find yourself reading your note cards too much, this is a sure clue you need to reduce the amount of written text on each card. Remember, all you need are short phrases or keywords, enough to "jog" your memory.

Use pictures or picture maps to guide you. Pictures help you to "visualise" the key points of your speech. Use mental pictures as well to tell the story in your head. This will take some creativity but will be worth the effort.

Using Visual Aids As Notes

Simple visual aids can effectively serve as headings and subheadings. Speak to the heading. Say what you want to say and move on. If you forget something, that's okay; the audience will never know unless you tell them.

Practice creating just a few meaningful headings to use and practice using only these headings as your "cues". This will take practice, but practising using only these few words will force you to better internalise your speech.

This has four important advantages:

You don't have to worry about what you are going to say next. Your visual aids provide you with your "cues" of your next major idea or thought. All you need to do between ideas is to use an effective transitional statement.

Having only a few keywords on your visual aid allows you to move around the room without the need or feeling you need to go back to your notes. In fact, most inexperienced speakers don't move around at all. The movement also helps you to relax and adds energy to your presentations.

The movement also allows the listeners to follow you and pay closer attention to you and your message. Plan your movements during your rehearsals. Decide where in your presentation it makes sense to move. If you find yourself starting to sway from side to side, take one or two steps and stop again, standing evenly on both feet. Keep your weight evenly distributed on both feet. This will help keep you from swaying.

You can have good eye contact with your audience. You can look at your audience all the time while speaking - except for that brief moment you look at your visual aid. But that's okay since the audience will probably follow you and also look at your visual aid.

This will help the audience to "see" your message as well as "hear" your message. The more you rehearse and the more you become familiar with your visual aids, the easier it becomes.

Your audience will feel comfortable that you are on your planned track. Well-designed visuals aids show the audience that you DO have a plan and have properly prepared and are following your plan.

Keep in mind; your visual aids do not have to be only word charts. They can contain diagrams, pictures or even graphs.

When you use visual aids, always introduce the visual aid BEFORE you show it using one of your transition statements. You can even use the "looking back / looking forward" transition: "Now that we have seen the ...let's now look at...."

Regardless of which method you choose to use to remember your material, nothing will help you more than proper planning and preparation. Remember to prepare, prepare, prepare!

Movie quote...

"Everybody gets one chance to do something great." THE SANDLOT

When Benny can't psych himself up to face the Beast, we all felt for him. Our own Beasts scare us every day. When we get our one chance, to do a dream speech.

Hints for Eliminating Verbal Clutter

These tips will help you become more aware of your speaking manner:

Before you begin to speak, think about the words you want to use.

Think about what you want to say before you open your mouth.

When you find yourself saying uhs and ums (verbal clutter), stop yourself and repeat the sentence, this time replacing the ahs and ums with silence.

Use the pause as an effective technique. Work hard at replacing this verbal clutter with a simple pause, and during these short pauses allow your mind to catch up and think about what you want to say next.

Practice some of these quick tricks in everyday speaking situations such as making a phone call or running into someone at a bank or store, but this time focus on replacing your verbal clutter with silence.

How To Cure The Verbal Virus

A Five-Step Treatment Plan

Verbal viruses are meaningless fillers that speckle our speech, distract from our message, drain our impact and annoy listeners.

The most common verbal viruses are: "uh" "um" "like" "you know" "well" "okay" and "sort of". They also include annoying mouth sounds and lip smacks.

Verbal viruses are jarring to the ear and inconsistent with a professional image. They can make you sound unsure, unprepared and poorly educated. The good news about verbal viruses is that they are easily cured.

1. Diagnose The Problem: Since verbal viruses are unconscious, the only way you'll hear them is on tape. Record a few of your phone calls on a typical business day to quickly determine if you are suffering from a verbal virus infection.

2. Pause: Whenever you catch yourself saying a non-word, just stop talking. Say nothing. This gap of silence will feel scary at first, but if the pause is no longer than 5 seconds, the listener will scarcely notice. A pause will help you gather your thoughts while giving the listener time to reflect on what you have just said.

3. Record The Voicemail Messages You Leave For Others: Listen to them at the end of the day and note whether or not unwanted fillers have crept into your messages.

4. Enlist The Help Of A Friend Or Partner: Explain what you are trying to do and invent a code word he or she can use every time you use a filler word. The constant reminder will help you break the habit fast.

5. Hold Your Breath. When you feel you are about to use a non-word, take a breath, hold it for a moment and then begin to speak. The focus on your breathing will occupy your mind, keep you calm and centred and make the silence between the words seem much less scary.

Teach Self Hypnosis

Methods of self-hypnosis range from listening to relaxation tapes to simply clearing your mind of thoughts and worries. Here is a step-by-step free guide to self-hypnosis, using one approach you may find helpful. I encourage clients to learn self-hypnosis.

Please note that self-hypnosis should never be practised when driving, operating machinery or carrying out any other activity that requires your full attention.

What do you want to achieve?

Always be clear and specific about your goals and write them down before you begin your hypnosis. Writing down what it is you want to achieve or change can really help you to straighten things out in your mind and goals can suddenly look more realistic, specific and focused. Keep it short and keep it achievable. Stick to one or two goals only in a single session.

Write out a plan

Plan what you want to say from beginning to end. You can write out a detailed script to follow as part of your preparation.

Repeat your goals

Write several different suggestions for each goal, expressing the same goal in different ways. This will reinforce the suggestion and ensure that it is accepted into the unconscious mind.

Create your own vision for your success

Develop your own imagery and symbols for supporting and visualising your goals. Imagine yourself achieving whatever you wish to. Make it real, like a memory but in the future.

Make it personal

Use language and images which reflect your own experience. We all have our own memories and experiences of the world and speak to ourselves in our own language. Put your suggestions into your own words and use images you are familiar with.

Use your voice

Begin the session in your normal voice at a relaxed pace. As the session progresses, slow down and soften your voice so that as you enter hypnosis, you are speaking softly, and at a slower pace than when you began. Your voice can return to normal at the end of the session as you leave hypnosis.

Make yourself comfortable

Find a place that is quiet, comfortable and free from disturbance to practice self-hypnosis. You certainly must not be driving or in any other situation where your immediate attention is required. Soft music and lighting may help but we would not recommend the burning of candles.

Relax

Use deep breathing and relaxation techniques to prepare for entering hypnosis. Just focus internally and start to notice whatever you notice. This is not a time for judging, analysing, criticising or worrying. Notice your thoughts and feelings and assume that very soon they will just drift away - they are really not necessary at the moment. Allow your mind to become calmer and clearer.

Count yourself down

Use 'deepeners' in your hypnosis script, such as going down a staircase or an elevator, or floating down a stream, to help yourself go deeper into your hypnosis. Countdown in your mind as you go deeper into relaxation. At times there will be inner resistance to relaxation especially when you first start to practice self-hypnosis. Just be aware of it and let it go...It will!

Create an inner world

Spend some time in your own special place. Create your own magical place in your mind, maybe somewhere you know, maybe just an imagined paradise. This can be a place where you feel safe and relaxed and anything is possible. Use all of your senses - what can you see, hear, feel, smell and taste? Make this experience as vivid as you can, again, you will get much better with practice.

Make it easier next time

Towards the end of your trance, include some post-hypnotic suggestions for re-entering self-hypnosis next time you practice.

Count yourself back

At the end of your session, count yourself back to full awareness. Suggest to yourself that when you leave hypnosis you will feel refreshed and alert. Check that you are once again fully awake and alert and enjoy the rest of the day!

Dealing with difficult participants

The Heckler –

Probably insecure

Aggressive and argumentative

Gets satisfaction from needing

What to do –

Never get upset

Wait for a misstatement of fact and then throw it out to the group

Find merit, express agreement on something, move on

The Griper –

Will use you as a scapegoat

Feels 'hard done by'

Probably has a pet 'peeve'

What to do –

Use peer pressure

Get him/her to be specific

Show that the purpose of your presentation is to be positive and constructive

The Talker / Know all

Well-informed and anxious to show it

An 'eager beaver'/ chatterbox

A show-off

What to do –

Jump in and ask for the group to comment

Use as a 'co-presenter' – maybe he/she has some interesting points to add

Wait till he/she takes a breath, thank, refocus and move on

Slow him/her down with a tough question

The Whisperers –

Don't understand what's going on – clarifying or translating

Bored, mischievous or hypercritical

Sharing anecdotes triggered by your presentation

What to do –

Stop taking, wait for them to look up and 'non-verbally' ask for their permission to continue

Stare at them in silence, until everyone is looking at them

Remember that questions are not always questions, just a chance to show

QUESTION & ANSWER TIME

Reflect back to the questioner what you thought was the question;

(If I understand correctly, you're asking....)

Deflect it as follows:

Group - How do you the rest of the group feel?

- Has anyone else had a similar problem?

Ricochet – (to one participant) "John, you're an expert on this?

Reverse – (Back to questioner) "You've obviously done some thinking on this, what's your view?

Answer the question

Do a demo with the person who asked the question

Personal reference

Who is the most qualified person to answer this question

Don't answer the question

Relevancy challenge – it's outside the framework

Hold on to the question, answer it later on

Listen and pass it on

So if you were in my position – How would you answer it – listen to move on

I have never heard the question asked like that before

When it goes wrong …. Be prepared for these

Forced attendance

Dismissive gesture

Disagreement

Boredom

Distraction

Takes offence

Refusal to do exercise

The demo doesn't work

High jacking

Conflict among participants

Beliefs violated

Jokers

Skill levels

The above list is things just to be prepared for when doing your presentation. We have discussed many ways of dealing with all of the above in the book. Plus ask your unconscious mind in self-hypnosis.

Preparation is the key – Be prepared to be attacked

Additional Tips on Handling Questions

A. Ask people to stand up when they ask a question. This does two things:

(1) It shows you more readily who is asking the question, and (2) It makes it easier for the audience to also hear the question.

B. Have small sheets of paper available for people to write down their questions during your presentation. They may forget what they were going to ask earlier.

C. Allow people to pass the questions to you if they feel uncomfortable standing up and asking the question out loud. This gives the person who truly wants to ask a question an option.

D. Always repeat the question - this does three things:

(1) It makes sure you understood the question, (2) It gives you a chance to value the question and think of an answer, (3) It assures the other people in the audience can hear the question since you are facing them.

E. Always take time to think "before" you answer all questions. This allows you time to think, especially for those difficult questions.

Do the same for those questions you readily know the answer for.

Responding too quickly to those questions you are most comfortable with will only bring attention to those questions you do not.

F. Have a pencil and paper available for you to write down questions you can't answer. You select someone to record the questions on paper.

This way, you can properly follow up with the person who asked the question you couldn't answer. Be sure to get their name & phone number or address. Promise to get back to them and DO get back to them.

Remember:

The presentation starts when you arrive, make yourself available, all the time you are there.

If you're not sure where you're going, you'll probably end up somewhere else.

- unknown

Anxiety (How to remove)

Past   Now   Future

Presentation Day

Procedure:

1. "Float up above the Time Line, and out into the future to 15 minutes after the successful completion of the event about which you thought you were anxious. Tell me when you're there/"

2. "Good. Turn and look toward now/ along the Time Line."

3. "Now, where's the anxiety?"

4. "Come back to now."

5. If desired/ test by having them think about what used to make them anxious, and notice that the feeling is emotionally balanced/ or flat.

NOTE: If anxiety does not disappear, then reframe, "I know that there's a part of you that thinks it's important for you to have some anxiety to motivate you, and I agree that it's important for you to be motivated.

The problem is that anxiety is not good for the body. Are there other ways that would be OK for you to motivate yourself, and let the anxiety go?"

Top Ten Tips for Presenting

Don't try and win the Nobel prize for technical accuracy

Use humour, a laugh is worth a thousand frowns

Exaggerate body movements and verbal emphasis

Don't keep your eyes on your notes

Never read anything except quotations

If you are not nervous there's something wrong

Pause often – silence is much longer for you than for the audience

Keep it simple

Be enthusiastic – if you're not, why should they be

Perform (don't act)

Overlapping metaphors

NLP Overlapping Representational Systems Script

When a person has trouble accessing a representational sy1stem, they are limited in the way they recall memories, assign meaning and interact with the world. The problem often results from trauma, but can also be a result of an underdeveloped representational system. This technique will help them in developing access to that system.

Identify the underrepresented modality

For example, if someone were unable to access pictures in their mind (created or remembered), but wanted to be able to do visualization exercises or just wanted to be able to make pictures, we would work on the Visual representational system.

Begin with the favoured representational system

Begin helping the client to create strong I/Rs in their preferred system.

For example:

Just imagine yourself in a wonderfully majestic forest...

a.   Visual: You can see the leaves gently moving in the breeze as the moon begins rising above the trees in the distance. You see a small brook nearby, and the water twists lazily through its random course.

b. Auditory: You can hear the wind blowing through the big leaves on the full trees, hear the crickets in the background, and hear a babbling brook lazily drifting by in the distance.

c. Kinesthetic: You can feel the gentle wind blowing, feeling the soft ground beneath your feet, and being in this forest makes you feel so peaceful.

Then overlap to the underrepresented system

Examples:

Visual to Auditory: And as you see these things, you can begin to hear the gentle rustling of the leaves in the trees that surround you.

Kinesthetic to Visual: And as you feel those things, you begin noticing the rich colour of the leaves on all trees around you.

Auditory to Kinesthetic: And as you hear those sounds around, you begin to feel a sense of calm as it envelops you in the warm, gentle breeze.

Test

Think of a happy memory from your past, and describe to me what it (looked/sounded/felt) like.

Future Pace

As you think about your future, think of a time when having access to this part of your mind will help you be successful. Describe that to me.

Swish Pattern

NLP Swish Pattern 1: Identify the Problem Behaviour

Before you use the NLP Swish Pattern, you have to know which problem behaviour you are looking to change.

This could be – you don't exercise enough, you eat too much crap – or it could be a fear of meeting new people, of speaking in public, or a fear of failing at any particular endeavour.

All that matters is that it's an exact behaviour that you would like to change – to replace with a new positive and empowering response.

Pick a specific problem you are looking to solve with the NLP Swish Pattern before you move on.

NLP Swish Pattern 2: Find The Cue

Your current problem behaviour is likely to be triggered automatically by a specific stimulus. This means that you don't consciously choose to act the way you do, you just do. It's an automatic response - just like when the Doctor bangs your knee with a hammer and your leg shoots up.

There is a certain trigger for you that causes you to act out this problem behaviour. If you can identify the trigger, you can change the response with an NLP Swish Pattern.

For example, if you're putting off going to the gym, what is the exact moment that you decide not to go? It could be the thought of packing your bag and walking to the gym that makes you decide against it.

It might be the mental image of you struggling on the running machine that saps your enthusiasm. It could even be the "better" thought of you lying on the sofa, junk food and TV remote in hand, as a preferred way to spend your afternoon.

Either way, there is a specific cue that generates an automatic response. Find this before moving on.

If you're struggling to identify your specific cue, try this little exercise – imagine that you have to teach me this problem behaviour.

Imagine that I want to learn how to avoid exercise, or how to eat more crap, or how to be petrified of speaking in public – or whatever your particular issue is.

What is the one image that I would need to picture that would absolutely decide my hand for me? Which pictures, sounds and feelings would I have to replicate in my brain to confine me to acting out the undesired response? If you really, truly wanted to convince me why you act the way you do, how would you do so? What do I need to see and feel to make me act this way?

That should've helped you to find your trigger! If you haven't identified your cue yet, simply imagine performing your now... what pops into your mind first? How do you manage to convince yourself that this better and more beneficial behaviour is a bad or scary idea?

When you've identified your cue, jot it down on a bit of paper and break state – this simply means clearing your brain and doing something else for a few seconds. Jump up and down on the spot, hum a song, recite the alphabet backwards or look out the window for a while...

Whatever you fancy. Just think about something totally unrelated for a minute before proceeding. This helps your brain to reset before you go on to identify the new behaviour you wish to install.

NLP Swish Pattern 3: Choose Your Ideal Response

Now we get to the fun part. Here, you get to choose the self-image that you will install in your subconscious – the positive response you will generate automatically when the cue occurs from now on.

Choose a suitably compelling snapshot of you performing at your best now – a picture that excites and motivates you.

For example, you might see yourself immediately after a gym session - buzzing on endorphins and feeling wonderful. You might imagine a slim and healthy you who is eating healthily and feeling awesome. It could be confident and assured you who has just delivered an engaging and well-received presentation to a crowd of strangers and received rapturous applause. Whatever the response you wish to install, get a clear picture of it now.

All that matters is that this response is powerful for you – it has to motivate you and you only.

Now... ramp it up! Make the picture big and bright and gorgeously compelling... make the sounds brighter and clearer... and thoroughly indulge yourself in every last glorious detail of this wonderful picture... and make sure you feel exactly how you would feel if you acted in this ideal way in real life... better, in fact.

Now, locate where the feeling in your body is, give this feeling a colour, and double its intensity and brightness... and then double it again! Make yourself feel awesome now by seeing yourself performing at your best – and living it now in the present.

Absolutely wallow in this gorgeous collection of images, sounds and feelings. Make yourself feel as amazing as you possibly can... and then double the intensity of the feelings again! Make sure your brain is filled with a gloriously bright, crisp and powerful image of you at your best – and feeling on top of the world.

When you've got this wonderful image sorted, break state. Count to ten in Japanese. Converse with a pet. Contemplate the nature of the universe... whatever takes your fancy.

NLP Swish Pattern 4: Time To Swish!

This is where the magic happens! What you are going to do is take the original cue image from step 2 and replace it with the new, empowering picture from step 3.

So first, get the old cue picture in your mind. You should be associated – which means seeing it through your own eyes. Make it big and bright and see every little detail.

Now, take a postage-stamp sized picture of your new, powerful self-image, and plonk it in the corner of your vision. Make it small and dark and disassociated for the moment – which means looking down at yourself from a third party perspective, not through your own eyes.

Now, we're ready to Swish!

Take the postage sized picture of the new you and push it further and further away from you until it is just a tiny speck. I like to visualise this little picture stretching all the way back to the moon, where I load it with an unimaginably powerful rocket launcher.

(In a second we're going to need this image to absolutely fly at you, growing bigger and brighter and more compelling by the millisecond – and I find the best way to do this is by imagining the new picture has a rocket strapped to it. Some people prefer pretending it's on an elastic band – work out what's right for you!)

When you're ready to Swish, fire your rocket or elastic band at full power. As the new image comes hurtling towards you, becoming bigger and richer and bolder – send the old cue image in the opposite direction, armed with its very own rocket launcher, making it darker and smaller and less powerful and flying away from you.

Some people like to make an audible "Swish" sound when they do this – I guess it's the sound you'd imagine these memories to make as they fly past each other.

As the new self-image hits you – associate. See it through your own eyes! Imagine every last glorious detail again and make it big and bright and bold and beautiful! Feel all the amazing feelings rush through your veins... And think how good it would be to behave like this from now on.

Take a few moments to revel in the wonderful feeling of this new self-image. This is key – indulge yourself. Don't rush this bit... enjoy your success.

Now, break state.

NLP Swish Pattern 5: Embed The Change

It's now time to thoroughly embed this change. For the NLP Swish Pattern to work, you need to repeat the last step 10 times, breaking state in between each one. You'll find that you'll do this quickly as you progress.

(Don't moan! It will only take you ten minutes tops – and if you've come this far, it's bloody worth it!)

So, load up the old cue image – put the new empowering belief as a speck in the corner – push it back as far as it can go - load it up with your rocket or spring – and Swish! Send the old memory to the moon, and bring the new memory crushing home to you!

Take a few moments between each attempt to really enjoy the feelings... you should be having fun when you do this.

To finish, when you have Swished 10 times, think of the cue and then try and think of your old problem behaviour. If you've done it correctly, it will be quite tricky to even imagine the old behaviour – and even if you can, it's most probably lost the majority of its strength. You might even find it a bit funny to imagine yourself behaving in the old way... Success!

You're now left with a new way to act whenever you experience the cue – so enjoy the results from this NLP Swish Pattern!

Exercise:- Final Presentation

Position 1 – Presenter

Position 2 – Audience member

Position 3 – Observer of presenter

Do a presentation for 5 minutes

Now Step to third, what can be improved

Step back to 1st with improvements

Continue presentation for another 5 minutes

Back to 3rd - gives feel back to 1st position

Integrate

Position 3 Questions

Q - What specifically you liked?

Q – What specifically can be improved?

11 Tips for Using Flip Charts More Effectively

While everyone seems to be interested in creating high-tech computer-generated presentations, the flip chart still continues to be the most effective presentation media of all. One should not assume that investing a lot of money in high tech visual aids & equipment will "make" your presentation.

The best visuals have been and still are the simplest. Remember, the purpose of using visual aids is to enhance your presentation, not upstage it.

Since most presentations are delivered before small groups of 35 people or less, the flip chart is a perfect size. I feel the flip chart will continue to be the workhorse of most training seminars.

There are several advantages of using a flip chart. Here are just a few:

Flip charts do not need electricity - You don't need to worry if the bulb will burn out or worry that you forgot the extension cord.

Flip charts are economical - They do not require you to use any special films or printers to produce them.

Colour can be added very easily - An inexpensive box of flip chart markers allows you all the creativity you want.

Flip charts allow spontaneity - Any last minute changes can be easily made.

In today's world of high tech computers, fancy software and sophisticated infomercials, many presenters today feel they have to create a presentation which shows off their ability to use computers and their latest clip art library.

Although the software available today does allow everyone the ability to create colourful slides and overheads, we often find that the visuals become the presentation and not the speaker. As a speaker, your visual aids should not be the presentation. You are!

Even though flip charts are low tech, they are reliable and don't require any special skill to use them but here are some tips to help you use them effectively.

1. The best flip chart stands have clamps at the top and will hold the most type of flip chart pads. Most allow you to hang your flip charts while some stands will only allow you to prop them up. Don't wait until the last minute to find this out.

2. Make sure the flip charts you use will fit the flip chart stand you will be using. Some have different spaced holes at the top.

3. Flipchart pads are usually sold in packages of two and come either plain or with grid lines on them. Using the pad with grid lines makes your job easier for drawing straight lines and keeps your text aligned. Also, make sure the pad has perforations at the top to allow easier removal of sheets. Many presenters struggle to tear off a sheet evenly.

4. When preparing your charts, it is best to first design your charts on paper first before drawing them on the actual flip chart pad.

5. Lightly write your text in pencil first before using the actual flip chart markers. This will allow you to make any adjustments with text spacing and any figures you will be drawing. Do NOT use all block letters (UPPERCASE). Using upper and lower case letters makes it easier to read. I like to use the 7 x 7 rule. Have no more than 7 words on each line and no more than 7 lines to a sheet. Using a 6 x 6 rule is even better.

6. Use flip chart markers and not regular magic markers. Flip chart markers will not "bleed" through the paper. Also, they do not have as strong a smell as regular markers. You can also find "scented" markers. They usually come in various fruit scents.

7. Avoid using the colours yellow, pink, or orange. These are extremely difficult for the audience to see. Don't make your audience have to strain their eyes to see your points.

Avoid using too many colours. Using one dark colour and one accent colour works best.

8. You can write "lightly in pencil" any notes next to key points you need. The audience won't be able to see them. You may also write what is on the next sheet. Knowing this will allow you to properly introduce your next sheet.

9. If you make any mistakes you can use "white out" to correct any small errors. For larger areas, cover the mistake with a double layer of flip chart paper and correct the error.

10. Have a blank sheet of paper between each of your text sheets. This will prevent the written material from other sheets to "peek" through.

11. Properly store and transport your flip charts in a case or the cardboard box that some come in. This will protect your flip charts and keep them fresh and ready to use each time. Take great care of your flip charts.

Making "prepared" flip charts can take a considerable amount of time. Make sure you start preparing your charts early enough so you can review them and make any changes or corrections beforehand.

It takes practice to learn how to print neatly. If you do not have neat printing, ask someone who does prepare him or her for you. A poorly prepared flip chart can be very ugly.

Movie quote...

"You only have 16 minutes left in a Wildcats uniform, so make it count."

HIGH SCHOOL MUSICAL

The Wildcats make a habit of turning basketball into something that makes everyone want to jump into action with their catchy songs. But this speech right before the opening number of HSM 3 applies to more than the struggle between singing and sports. Remember this speech when you need to make your mark on a presentation.

Impromptu Speaking

While many of us do not like to speak in front of people, there are times when we are asked to get up and say a few words about someone or a topic when we have not planned on saying anything at all. We are more shocked than anyone else. Has this ever happened to you? If and when this does happen to you, be prepared to rise to the challenge.

Below are some tips you can use the next time you are called on to speak.

Decide quickly what your one message will be - Keep in mind you have not been asked to give a speech but to make some impromptu remarks. Hopefully, they have asked you early enough so you can at least jot down a few notes before you speak. If not, pick ONE message or comment and focus on that one main idea. Many times, other ideas may come to you after you start speaking. If this happens, go with the flow and trust your instincts.

Do not try and memorise what you will say - Trying to memorise will only make you more nervous and you will find yourself thinking more about the words and not about the message.

Start off strong and with confidence - If you at least plan your opening statement, this will get you started on the right foot. After all, just like with any formal speech, getting started is the most difficult. Plan what your first sentence will be. You may even write this opening line down on your note card and glance at it one more time just before you begin speaking.

If you know you have three points or ideas to say, just start off simple by saying, "I would just like to talk about 3 points". The first point is... the second point is... and so on.

Decide on your transitions from one point to the other - After you have decided on your opening remark or line, come up with a simple transition statement that takes you to your main point.

If you have more than one point to make, you can use a natural transition such as, "My second point is... or my next point is..." etc. Just list on your note card or napkin, if you have to, the main points or ideas.

Do not write out the exact words, but just the points you want to mention.

Maintain eye contact with the audience - This is easier to do if you do not write down all kinds of stuff to read. Look down at your next idea or thought and maintain eye contact with your audience and speak from your heart. Focus on communicating with your audience and not speaking AT the crowd.

Occasionally throw in an off-the-cuff remark - Because you want your style to be flexible and seem impromptu, trust your instinct and add a few words which just pop into your head. Keep it conversational and think of the audience as a group of your friends.

Finally, have a good conclusion - Gracefully just state, "And the last point I would like to make is ....". Once you have made your last point, you can then turn control back to the person who asked you to speak in the first place.

With a little practice, this process will feel more natural to you. Anticipating that you MAY be asked to say a few words should force you to at least think about what you might say if you are asked. Then if you ARE asked, you are better prepared because you anticipated being asked.

This is much better than thinking they won't ask you and they actually do!

"To accomplish great things, we must not only act but also dream; not only plan but also believe".

Understanding/overcoming fear

The key to managing and controlling anything is first to understand it, especially its causes.

The cause of fear is (a feeling of) insecurity and/or an unfamiliar or uncontrollable threat.

In the context of presentations and public speaking, this is usually due to:

• lack of confidence, and/or

• lack of control (or a feeling of not having control) - over the situation, other people (the audience) and our own reactions and feelings

• and (in some cases) possibly a bad memory or experience from our past

The effects of these are heightened according to the size of the audience, and potentially also the nature of the audience/situation - which combines to represent a perceived uncontrollable threat to us at a very basic and instinctive level (which we imagine in the form or critical judgment, embarrassment, humiliation, etc).

This 'audience' aspect is illustrated by the following:

"Most of us would not feel very fearful if required to give a presentation to a class of 30 five-year-old children, but we would feel somewhat more fearful if required to give a presentation to an interview panel of three high court judges. So audience size is not everything - it's the nature of the situation and audience too."

As such audience, size and situation are circumstantial factors which can influence the degree of anxiety, but they are not causal factors in themselves. The causes exist because of the pressure to command, control, impress, etc.

Confidence and control

The two big causal factors (low confidence and control) stem typically from:

- inadequate preparation/rehearsal, and/or

- low experience.

If we have a bad memory which is triggering a fear response, then it is likely that the original situation we recall, and which prompts our feelings of anxiety, resulting from one or both of the above factors.

Preparation and rehearsal are usually very manageable elements. It's a matter of making the effort to prepare and rehearse before the task is upon us. Presentations which do not work well usually do so because they have not been properly prepared and rehearsed.

Experience can be gained simply by seeking opportunities for public speaking and presenting to people and groups, wherever you feel most comfortable (and then try speaking to groups where you feel less comfortable).

Given that humankind and society everywhere are arranged in all sorts of groups - schools and colleges, evening classes, voluntary groups, open-mic nights, debating societies, public meetings, conferences, the local pub, sports and hobby clubs, hospitals, old people's homes, etc, etc - there are countless groups everywhere of people and potential audiences by which you can gain speaking and presenting experience - this is not so difficult to achieve.

So experience, is actually just another manageable element before the task, although more time and imagination is required than in preparing and rehearsing a particular presentation.

Besides these preparatory points, it's useful to consider that fear relates to stress.

Stress can be managed in various ways. Understanding stress and stress management methods can be very helpful in reducing the anxiety we feel before and while giving presentations and public speaking.

Physiology, chemistry, stress

Fear of public speaking is strongly related to stress.

A common physical reaction in people when having to speak in public is a release of adrenaline and cortisol into our systems, which is sometimes likened to drinking several cups of coffee. Even experienced speakers feel their heart thumping very excitedly indeed.

This sensational reaction to speaking in public is certainly not only felt by novices, and even some of the great professional actors and entertainers suffer from real physical sickness before taking the stage or podium.

So you are not alone. Speaking in public is genuinely scary for most people, including many who outwardly seem very calm.

Our primitive brain shuts down normal functions as the 'fight or flight' impulse takes over.

But don't worry - every person in your audience wants you to succeed. The audience is on your side (if only because they are very pleased that it's you up there in the spotlight speaking and not them).

The toughest part of getting to the top of the ladder is getting through the crowd at the bottom.

- Unknown

Apple founder Steve Jobs died on Wednesday, aged 56. In 2005, in a moving address at Stanford University after receiving surgery for pancreatic cancer, he reflected on his own mortality, urging his audience:

'Your time is limited, so don't waste it living someone else's life.'

Below is the full text from the speech

I am honoured to be with you today at your commencement from one of the finest universities in the world. I never graduated from college. Truth be told, this is the closest I've ever gotten to a college graduation. Today I want to tell you three stories from my life. That's it. No big deal. Just three stories.

The first story is about connecting the dots. I dropped out of Reed College after the first 6 months, but then stayed around as a drop-in for another 18 months or so before I really quit. So why did I drop out? It started before I was born. My biological mother was a young, unwed college graduate student, and she decided to put me up for adoption. She felt very strongly that I should be adopted by college graduates, so everything was all set for me to be adopted at birth by a lawyer and his wife.

Except that when I popped out they decided at the last minute that they really wanted a girl. So my parents, who were on a waiting list, got a call in the middle of the night asking: "We have an unexpected baby boy; do you want him?" They said: "Of course." My biological mother later found out that my mother had never graduated from college and that my father had never graduated from high school. She refused to sign the final adoption papers.

She only relented a few months later when my parents promised that I would someday go to college. And 17 years later I did go to college. But I naively chose a college that was almost as expensive as Stanford, and all of my working-class parents' savings were being spent on my college tuition. After six months, I couldn't see the value in it. I had no idea what I wanted to do with my life and no idea how college was going to help me figure it out. And here I was spending all of the money my parents had saved their entire life. So I decided to drop out and trust that it would all work out OK.

It was pretty scary at the time, but looking back it was one of the best decisions I ever made. The minute I dropped out I could stop taking the required classes that didn't interest me, and begin dropping in on the ones that looked interesting. It wasn't all romantic.

I didn't have a dorm room, so I slept on the floor in friends' rooms, I returned coke bottles for the 5¢ deposits to buy food with, and I would walk the seven miles across town every Sunday night to get one good meal a week at the Hare Krishna temple.

I loved it. And much of what I stumbled into by following my curiosity and intuition turned out to be priceless later on. Let me give you one example: Reed College at that time offered perhaps the best calligraphy instruction in the country. Throughout the campus, every poster, every label on every drawer, was beautifully hand calligraphed.

Because I had dropped out and didn't have to take the normal classes, I decided to take a calligraphy class to learn how to do this. I learned about serif and san serif typefaces, about varying the amount of space between different letter combinations, about what makes great typography great. It was beautiful, historical, artistically subtle in a way that science can't capture, and I found it fascinating. None of this had even a hope of any practical application in my life. But ten years later, when we were designing the first Macintosh computer, it all came back to me. And we designed it all into the Mac.

It was the first computer with beautiful typography. If I had never dropped in on that single course in college, the Mac would have never had multiple typefaces or proportionally spaced fonts. And since Windows just copied the Mac, it's likely that no personal computer would have them. If I had never dropped out, I would have never dropped in on this calligraphy class, and personal computers might not have the wonderful typography that they do.

Of course, it was impossible to connect the dots looking forward when I was in college. But it was very, very clear looking backwards ten years later. Again, you can't connect the dots looking forward; you can only connect them looking backwards. So you have to trust that the dots will somehow connect in your future. You have to trust in something — your gut, destiny, life, karma, whatever.

This approach has never let me down, and it has made all the difference in my life. My second story is about love and loss. I was lucky — I found what I loved to do early in life. Woz and I started Apple in my parent's garage when I was 20. We worked hard, and in 10 years Apple had grown from just the two of us in a garage into a $2bn company with over 4,000 employees.

We had just released our finest creation — the Macintosh — a year earlier, and I had just turned 30. And then I got fired. How can you get fired from a company you started? Well, as Apple grew we hired someone whom I thought was very talented to run the company with me, and for the first year or so things went well. But then our visions of the future began to diverge and eventually we had a falling out. When we did, our board of directors sided with him.

So at 30, I was out. And very publicly out. What had been the focus of my entire adult life was gone, and it was devastating. I really didn't know what to do for a few months. I felt that I had let the previous generation of entrepreneurs down - that I had dropped the baton as it was being passed to me.

I met with David Packard and Bob Noyce and tried to apologise for screwing up so badly. I was a very public failure, and I even thought about running away from the valley. But something slowly began to dawn on me — I still loved what I did. The turn of events at Apple had not changed that one bit. I had been rejected, but I was still in love. And so I decided to start over. I didn't see it then, but it turned out that getting fired from Apple was the best thing that could have ever happened to me.

The heaviness of being successful was replaced by the lightness of being a beginner again, less sure about everything. It freed me to enter one of the most creative periods of my life.

During the next five years, I started a company named NeXT, another company named Pixar, and fell in love with an amazing woman who would become my wife. Pixar went on to create the worlds first computer animated feature film, Toy Story and is now the most successful animation studio in the world. In a remarkable turn of events, Apple bought NeXT, I returned to Apple, and the technology we developed at NeXT is at the heart of Apple's current renaissance. And Laurene and I have a wonderful family together.

I'm pretty sure none of this would have happened if I hadn't been fired from Apple. It was awful tasting medicine, but I guess the patient needed it. Sometimes life hits you in the head with a brick. Don't lose faith. I'm convinced that the only thing that kept me going was that I loved what I did. You've got to find what you love. And that is as true for your work as it is for your lovers.

Your work is going to fill a large part of your life, and the only way to be truly satisfied is to do what you believe is great work. And the only way to do great work is to love what you do. If you haven't found it yet, keep looking. Don't settle. As with all matters of the heart, you'll know when you find it. And, like any great relationship, it just gets better and better as the years roll on. So keep looking until you find it. Don't settle.

My third story is about death. When I was 17, I read a quote that went something like: "If you live each day as if it was your last, someday you'll most certainly be right."

It made an impression on me, and since then, for the past 33 years, I have looked in the mirror every morning and asked myself: "If today were the last day of my life, would I want to do what I am about to do today?" And whenever the answer has been "No" for too many days in a row, I know I need to change something.

Remembering that I'll be dead soon is the most important tool I've ever encountered to help me make the big choices in life. Because almost everything — all external expectations, all pride, all fear of embarrassment or failure - these things just fall away in the face of death, leaving only what is truly important. Remembering that you are going to die is the best way I know to avoid the trap of thinking you have something to lose. You are already naked.

There is no reason not to follow your heart. About a year ago I was diagnosed with cancer. I had a scan at 7:30 in the morning, and it clearly showed a tumour on my pancreas. I didn't even know what a pancreas was. The doctors told me this was almost certainly a type of cancer that is incurable, and that I should expect to live no longer than three to six months.

My doctor advised me to go home and get my affairs in order, which is doctor's code for prepare to die. It means to try to tell your kids everything you thought you'd have the next 10 years to tell them in just a few months. It means to make sure everything is buttoned up so that it will be as easy as possible for your family. It means to say your goodbyes. I lived with that diagnosis all day.

Later that evening I had a biopsy, where they stuck an endoscope down my throat, through my stomach and into my intestines, put a needle into my pancreas and got a few cells from the tumour. I was sedated, but my wife, who was there, told me that when they viewed the cells under a microscope the doctors started crying because it turned out to be a very rare form of pancreatic cancer that is curable with surgery. I had the surgery and I'm fine now.

This was the closest I've been to facing death, and I hope it's the closest I get for a few more decades. Having lived through it, I can now say this to you with a bit more certainty than when death was a useful but purely intellectual concept: No one wants to die.

Even people who want to go to heaven don't want to die to get there. And yet death is the destination we all share. No one has ever escaped it. And that is as it should be because death is very likely the single best invention of life. It is life's change agent. It clears out the old to make way for the new. Right now the new is you, but someday not too long from now, you will gradually become the old and be cleared away.

Sorry to be so dramatic, but it is quite true. Your time is limited, so don't waste it living someone else's life.

Don't be trapped by dogma — which is living with the results of other people's thinking. Don't let the noise of others' opinions drown out your own inner voice. And most important, have the courage to follow your heart and intuition.

They somehow already know what you truly want to become. Everything else is secondary. When I was young, there was an amazing publication called The Whole Earth Catalogue, which was one of the bibles of my generation. It was created by a fellow named Stewart Brand not far from here in Menlo Park, and he brought it to life with his poetic touch. This was in the late 1960s, before personal computers and desktop publishing, so it was all made with typewriters, scissors, and Polaroid cameras.

It was sort of like Google in paperback form, 35 years before Google came along: it was idealistic, and overflowing with neat tools and great notions. Stewart and his team put out several issues of The Whole Earth Catalogue, and then when it had run its course, they put out a final issue. It was the mid-1970s, and I was your age.

On the back cover of their final issue was a photograph of an early morning country road, the kind you might find yourself hitchhiking on if you were so adventurous. Beneath it was the words: "Stay Hungry. Stay Foolish." It was their farewell message as they signed off. Stay Hungry. Stay Foolish. And I have always wished that for myself. And now, as you graduate to begin anew, I wish that for you.

Stay Hungry. Stay Foolish.

Thank you all very much.

Steve Jobs

The Author:- Gary Sellors

Gary is a certified NLP Trainer, trained personally by Dr John Grinder (NLP Co-creator & Professor of Linguistics). Gary is a much sort after person in the business world, recognised and used by many top companies now, and therefore able to offer a whole range of skills to the development of people in the many businesses.

Gary is CIPD Qualified with an HR and Management background, Also a tutor for the London College of Clinical Hypnosis and a YMCA Personal Fitness Trainer. Along with good knowledge of Emotional Intelligence, Quantum Touch, Thought Field Therapy, Animal Healing, Reiki and EFT.

He has previously done training and developing with the likes of the CLRPG (Central London Retail Personnel Group) which includes the likes of Harrods, Marks & Spencer's, Harvey Nichol's, Elstree Film Studios, etc..

Using his experience and passion for the training and development of Directors / Managers and Sports Professionals at all levels. Including coaching top athletes on their mindset and helping them win British and European Gold medals.

He offers bespoke training in many areas for businesses and one to one coaching along with a massive range of therapy work, along with continuing his work on restoring Natural Eyesight, by working with the brain and a few simple exercises in retraining the eyes.

Gary Sellors can be reached at:-

E-mail :- wellbeingconsultant@hotmail.co.uk

Website:- www.garysellors.com

Other books on Amazon by Gary Sellors

My Silence is Broken

This unique workbook is for the many survivors of Sexual Abuse and Rape. My Silence is Broken, is designed for the many thousands of survivors, maybe yourself or you may know someone who has or is being affected by Sexual Violence. This unique workbook starts to give the survivors who have not yet told anyone a voice. Wellbeing Consultant, Gary Sellors, confronts the traumatic experiences that people rarely talk about and encourages people to work through the workbook themselves.

The exercises support survivors through suppressed anger, resentment, humiliation, guilt, blame and allows them to start to understand what and why it happen to them. It is always important to remember, it was never the survivor's fault and that they are not alone in this world. My Silence is Broken, really does want people to come forward with a voice, feel supported and listened too.

He offers excellent realistic and practical exercises that have been shown to work with the many clients affected by Sexual Abuse. This emotional and inspiring work was started long before the Operation Yewtree Police investigations in 2012. Dr Gary Sellors is passionate about the work that he does when working with children, adults or even animals that have been affected by violence and or traumatic sexual experiences over a short or very long time period.

This workbook can be done in any order, that is relevant to the person reading it, there are no timescales. It is important that the person reading this book does the work on their own, although if they feel comfortable, would be nice to share with a trusted friend, parent, partner or just anyone that needs the support. With this workbook and the focused exercises, you will discover, deeper meanings, thought-provoking insights leading to a different understanding of the experience you went through. Therefore, gaining newfound confidence, support, inner strength and that puts you back in control of your life and relationships.

June 2015. The BBC news reported that there were not enough therapeutic interventions being offered for people affected by Sexual Abuse, Rape and Child Exploitation.

This workbook is that offer of intervention help. For the winners of TIME, Magazine 2017. "The Silence Breakers 2017" having a voice. Supporting the #MeToo campaign 2017, The Truth Project 2018 and the work that has been done over the last 10 years.

www.garysellors.com

Other books on Amazon by Gary Sellors

The Winning Mindset For Achieving Weight Loss

Losing weight is the number one problem of obesity in the western world today. Gary Sellors has an amazing insight, excellent knowledge and experience in helping people lose weight and achieve The Winning Mind Set for achieving weight loss.

- How to lose 10 pounds in a week.
- Do you want to feel confident and achieve success?
- Learn to stop emotional eating and love yourself more.
- Would you like to kick-start your weight loss?
- The revolutionary Mind Set for health and weight loss.

Using Gary's advice and the latest proven scientific methods will automatically help you to start losing weight straight away as your mind and positive Mind Set change. You can use them, again and again, to make you feel happier about yourself as you go all the way to your reduced shape, size and weight.

Gary Sellors, Wellbeing Consultant, Author of the groundbreaking book. My Silence is Broken. Offers you a unique insight into losing weight without just running faster and eating lettuce. Gary uses methods that are proven to work with the mind and body with the help of a little science, along with offering great advice for building confidence and restoring your self-esteem.

Gary has worked with Gold medal winning athletes, who simply changed their mindset and success was guaranteed. His book is based on extensive experience and offers practical and realistic information which will lead to achieving weight loss. Which and will remove the stress of wondering what is the right method for you. This book will give you the answers and the confident mindset to achieve weight loss and have that thinner body you desire.

www.garysellors.com

The next book is currently being written and will be published in 2019 and will be about my work with animals and Animal Healing.

Love and Light

Gary